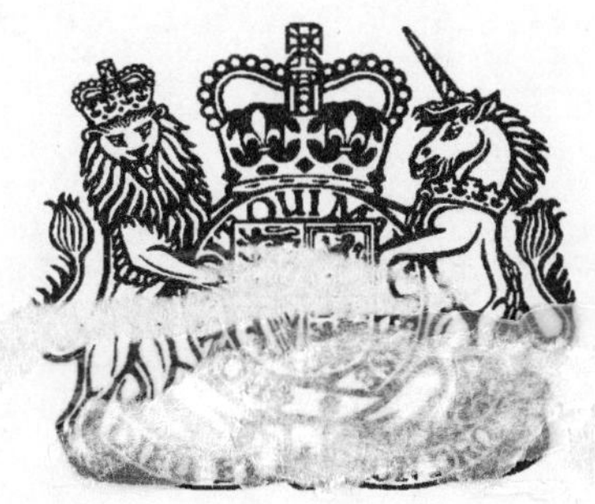

Carers and Disabled Children Act 2000

CHAPTER 16

ARRANGEMENT OF SECTIONS

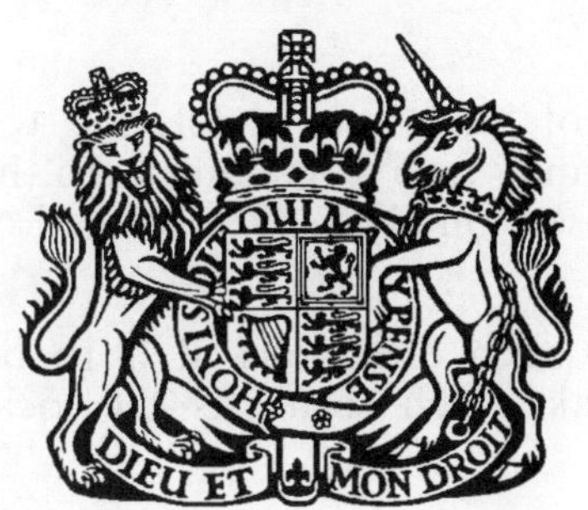

Carers and Disabled Children Act 2000

2000 CHAPTER 16

An Act to make provision about the assessment of carers' needs; to provide for services to help carers; to provide for the making of payments to carers and disabled children aged 16 or 17 in lieu of the provision of services to them; and for connected purposes.

[*20th July 2000*]

BE IT ENACTED by the Queen's most Excellent Majesty, by and with the advice and consent of the Lords Spiritual and Temporal, and Commons, in this present Parliament assembled, and by the authority of the same, as follows:—

1.—(1) If an individual aged 16 or over ("the carer")—

    (a) provides or intends to provide a substantial amount of care on a regular basis for another individual aged 18 or over ("the person cared for"); and

    (b) asks a local authority to carry out an assessment of his ability to provide and to continue to provide care for the person cared for,

the local authority must carry out such an assessment if it is satisfied that the person cared for is someone for whom it may provide or arrange for the provision of community care services.

(2) For the purposes of such an assessment, the local authority may take into account, so far as it considers it to be material, an assessment under section 1(1) of the Carers (Recognition and Services) Act 1995.

(3) Subsection (1) does not apply if the individual provides or will provide the care in question—

    (a) by virtue of a contract of employment or other contract with any person; or

    (b) as a volunteer for a voluntary organisation.

Right of carers to assessment.

1995 c. 12.

(4) The Secretary of State (or, in relation to Wales, the National Assembly for Wales) may give directions as to the manner in which an assessment under subsection (1) is to be carried out or the form it is to take.

(5) Subject to any such directions, it is to be carried out in such manner, and is to take such form, as the local authority considers appropriate.

(6) In this section, "voluntary organisation" has the same meaning as in the National Assistance Act 1948.

11 & 12 Geo. 6 c. 29.

Services for carers.

2.—(1) The local authority must consider the assessment and decide—

(a) whether the carer has needs in relation to the care which he provides or intends to provide;

(b) if so, whether they could be satisfied (wholly or partly) by services which the local authority may provide; and

(c) if they could be so satisfied, whether or not to provide services to the carer.

(2) The services referred to are any services which—

(a) the local authority sees fit to provide; and

(b) will in the local authority's view help the carer care for the person cared for,

and may take the form of physical help or other forms of support.

(3) A service, although provided to the carer—

(a) may take the form of a service delivered to the person cared for if it is one which, if provided to him instead of to the carer, could fall within community care services and they both agree it is to be so delivered; but

(b) if a service is delivered to the person cared for it may not, except in prescribed circumstances, include anything of an intimate nature.

(4) Regulations may make provision about what is, or is not, of an intimate nature for the purposes of subsection (3).

Vouchers.

3.—(1) Regulations may make provision for the issue of vouchers by local authorities.

(2) "Voucher" means a document whereby, if the local authority agrees with the carer that it would help him care for the person cared for if the carer had a break from caring, the person cared for may secure that services in lieu of the care which would otherwise have been provided to him by the carer are delivered temporarily to him by another person by way of community care services.

(3) The regulations may, in particular, provide—

(a) for the value of a voucher to be expressed in terms of money, or of the delivery of a service for a period of time, or both;

(b) for the person who supplies a service against a voucher, or for the arrangement under which it is supplied, to be approved by the local authority;

(c) for vouchers to be issued to the carer or to the person cared for;

(d) for a maximum period during which a service (or a service of a prescribed description) can be provided against a voucher.

4.—(1) In section 1 of the Carers (Recognition and Services) Act 1995 (which provides for carers to be assessed as to their ability to care in connection with an assessment of the needs of the individual cared for), after subsection (2) insert—

> "(2A) For the purposes of an assessment under subsection (1) or (2), the local authority may take into account, so far as it considers it to be material, an assessment under section 1 or 6 of the Carers and Disabled Children Act 2000."

(2) Subsection (4) applies if the local authority—

(a) is either providing services under this Act to the carer, or is providing community care services to or in respect of the person cared for (but not both); and

(b) proposes to provide another service to (or in respect of) the one who is not receiving any such service,

and the new service, or any service already being provided, is one which could be provided either under this Act, or by way of community care services.

(3) Subsection (4) also applies if—

(a) the local authority is not providing services to the carer (under this Act) or to the person cared for (by way of community care services), but proposes to provide services to each of them following an assessment under section 1 and under section 47 of the National Health Service and Community Care Act 1990; or

(b) the local authority is providing services both to the carer (under this Act) and to the person cared for (by way of community care services), and proposes to provide to either of them a new service,

and (in a paragraph (a) case) any of the services, or (in a paragraph (b) case) the new service, is one which could be provided either under this Act, or by way of community care services.

(4) In the case of each such service, the local authority must decide whether the service is, or is in future, to be provided under this Act, or by way of community care services (and hence whether it is, or is in future, to be provided to the carer, or to the person cared for).

(5) The local authority's decision under subsection (4) is to be made without regard to the means of the carer or of the person cared for.

5.   In section 1(1) of the Community Care (Direct Payments) Act 1996 (which provides for the making of payments for securing the provision of services which a person is assessed as needing)—

(a) in paragraph (a), at the end insert "or under section 2(1) of the Carers and Disabled Children Act 2000 (services for carers) to provide a person with services under that Act,";

Assessments and services for both carer and person cared for.
1995 c. 12.

1990 c. 19.

Direct payments.
1996 c. 30.

    (b) for paragraph (b), substitute—

        "(b) in the case of a person—

            (i) whose needs the local authority have decided call for the provision of community care services, he is of a description which is specified for the purposes of this subsection by regulations made by the Secretary of State, or

            (ii) whom the local authority have decided to provide with services under the Carers and Disabled Children Act 2000, he is not of a description so specified by regulations made by the Secretary of State,"; and

    (c) after "his needs call" insert "or, as the case may be, they have decided to provide (or arrange to provide)".

Assessments: persons with parental responsibility for disabled children.

6.—(1) If a person with parental responsibility for a disabled child—

    (a) provides or intends to provide a substantial amount of care on a regular basis for the child; and

    (b) asks a local authority to carry out an assessment of his ability to provide and to continue to provide care for the child,

the local authority must carry out such an assessment if it is satisfied that the child and his family are persons for whom it may provide or arrange for the provision of services under section 17 of the Children Act 1989 ("the 1989 Act").

1989 c. 41.

(2) For the purposes of such an assessment, the local authority may take into account, so far as it considers it to be material, an assessment under section 1(2) of the Carers (Recognition and Services) Act 1995.

1995 c. 12.

(3) The Secretary of State (or, in relation to Wales, the National Assembly for Wales) may give directions as to the manner in which an assessment under subsection (1) is to be carried out or the form it is to take.

(4) Subject to any such directions, it is to be carried out in such manner, and is to take such form, as the local authority considers appropriate.

(5) The local authority must take the assessment into account when deciding what, if any, services to provide under section 17 of the 1989 Act.

(6) Terms used in this section have the same meaning as in Part III of the 1989 Act.

Vouchers, and direct payments to disabled children and persons with parental responsibility for them.

7.—(1) In the Children Act 1989, after section 17 insert—

"Direct payments.

    17A.—(1) Instead of providing services in the exercise of functions conferred on them by section 17, a local authority may make to a person falling within subsection (2) (if he consents) a payment of such amount as, subject to subsections (5) and (6), they think fit in respect of his securing the provision of any of the services which the local authority would otherwise have provided.

    (2) The following fall within this subsection—

        (a) a person with parental responsibility for a disabled child;

(b) a disabled child aged 16 or 17.

(3) A payment under subsection (1) shall be subject to the condition that the person to whom it is made shall not secure the provision of the service to which it relates by a person who is of a prescribed description.

(4) The Secretary of State may by regulations provide that the power conferred by subsection (1) is not to be exercisable in relation to the provision of residential accommodation for any person for a period exceeding a prescribed period.

(5) Except as mentioned in subsection (6) of this section, subsections (2) and (6) of section 1, and subsections (1) and (2) of section 2, of the Community Care (Direct Payments) Act 1996 apply in relation to payments under subsection (1) as they apply in relation to payments under section 1(1) of that Act, but as if— 1996 c. 30.

(a) the reference to "subsection (4)" in section 1(6)(b) of that Act were a reference to subsection (3) of this section; and

(b) the references to "the relevant community care enactment" in section 2 of that Act were to Part III of the Children Act 1989. 1989 c. 41.

(6) Section 1(2) of the Community Care (Direct Payments) Act 1996 does not apply in relation to payments under subsection (1) to—

(a) a person with parental responsibility for a disabled child, other than a parent of such a child under the age of sixteen, in respect of a service which would otherwise have been provided for the child; or

(b) any person who is in receipt of income support, working families' tax credit or disabled person's tax credit under Part VII of the Social Security Contributions and Benefits Act 1992 or of an income-based jobseeker's allowance, 1992 c. 4.

and in those cases the amount of any payment under subsection (1) is to be at a rate equal to the local authority's estimate of the reasonable cost of securing the provision of the service concerned.

Vouchers for persons with parental responsibility for disabled children.

17B.—(1) The Secretary of State may by regulations make provision for the issue by a local authority of vouchers to a person with parental responsibility for a disabled child.

(2) "Voucher" means a document whereby, if the local authority agrees with the person with parental responsibility that it would help him care for the child if the person with parental responsibility had a break from caring, that person may secure the temporary provision of services for the child under section 17.

(3) The regulations may, in particular, provide—

    (a) for the value of a voucher to be expressed in terms of money, or of the delivery of a service for a period of time, or both;

    (b) for the person who supplies a service against a voucher, or for the arrangement under which it is supplied, to be approved by the local authority;

    (c) for a maximum period during which a service (or a service of a prescribed description) can be provided against a voucher."

1989 c. 41.
S.I. 1999/672.

(2) The reference to the Children Act 1989 in Schedule 1 to the National Assembly for Wales (Transfer of Functions) Order 1999 is to be treated as referring to that Act as amended by this section.

(3) Subsection (2) does not affect the power to make further Orders varying or omitting that reference.

Charging.
1983 c. 41.

8. In section 17 of the Health and Social Services and Social Security Adjudications Act 1983 (which provides for charges for local authority services in England and Wales), in subsection (2), after paragraph (e) insert—

    "(f) section 2 of the Carers and Disabled Children Act 2000".

Minor and consequential amendments.
1970 c. 42.
1996 c. 30.

9. In Schedule 1 to the Local Authority Social Services Act 1970 (which sets out enactments conferring functions referred to each local authority's social services committee)—

    (a) in the entry relating to the Community Care (Direct Payments) Act 1996, in the second column, at the end insert "or services under the Carers and Disabled Children Act 2000"; and

    (b) at the end, insert—

"Carers and Disabled Children Act 2000 (c. 16) The whole Act, in so far as it confers functions on a local authority within the meaning of that Act.	Assessment of carers' needs. Provision of services to carers. Provision of vouchers."

Financial provision.

10. There shall be paid out of money provided by Parliament any increase attributable to this Act in the sums payable out of money so provided by virtue of any other Act.

Interpretation and regulations.

11.—(1) Except as provided in section 6(6), in this Act—

"carer" and "person cared for" have the meaning given in section 1;

1990 c. 19.

"community care services" and "local authority" have the meaning given in section 46(3) of the National Health Service and Community Care Act 1990;

"prescribed" means prescribed in regulations; and

"regulations" means regulations made by statutory instrument by the Secretary of State (in relation to England) or by the National Assembly for Wales (in relation to Wales).